Alcoholism and its stages.

One of today's most popular product is alcohol. Alcoholic drinks of all types and grades are in demand by the vast majority of modern people, and each one way or another, consume alcohol. Only different types of beverages consumed, about their drinking and frequency of consumption.

Any alcoholic beverage includes a proportion of ethyl alcohol (it is indicated on the packaging), or ethanol with the chemical formula $C_2H_5(OH)$. Ethyl alcohol is a powerful neuroparalytic poison disrupts the functioning of the human nervous system and inflicting indelible damage to all groups of the internal organs of their customers. People voluntarily absorb the poison with or without - and often non-normalized consumption of alcoholic beverages leads to dangerous for the physical and mental health illness - alcoholism.

Alcoholism - a mental illness, excessive consumption of alcohol. As a result, permanent intoxication, a man greatly deteriorating health, decreases the ability to work, welfare and moral values. Alcoholism is characterized by the fact that a person becomes dependent on alcohol. So when there is no alcohol, alcoholic suffering and to ease their suffering, he repeats the reception of alcohol again and again. Alcoholism is not compatible with a healthy lifestyle.

Despite the debate among experts about whether to consider alcoholism a disease, the National Institute on Alcohol Abuse and Alcoholism recognize alcoholism as a disease. At the risk of developing alcoholism affect human genes and lifestyle behavior with regards to alcohol. Alcoholism is a chronic disease that lasts a lifetime. If you diagnose and treat it in its early stages, it is possible to cure and prevent serious complications. Chronic abuse of alcohol increases the risk of serious health problems such as liver disease, high blood pressure, heart disease, stroke, cancer (especially cancers of the esophagus, mouth and throat) and pancreatitis.

Alcoholism

About two million Russians suffer from liver damage caused by alcohol abuse. In 10 - 20% of drinkers will develop cirrhosis, which is characterized by scarring of the liver and causes irreversible damage. Cirrhosis leads to further deterioration of health and, ultimately, death. In addition to cirrhosis, heavy drinkers suffer from chronic liver disease and alcoholic hepatitis.

Liver damage causes problems with the level of blood sugar. When alcohol is present in the body, the liver processes it. Since the liver is busy metabolism of alcohol, it is often unable to maintain blood sugar at the appropriate level, which may lead to hypoglycemia (low blood sugar). When this happens, the brain is unable to obtain the necessary energy to function, and there are symptoms such as hunger, weakness, headache, tremor, and even coma (in severe cases).

Chronic alcohol abuse can lead to malnutrition. Chronic alcoholics not eat a sufficient amount of food because of the high caloric content of alcohol. It does not allow them to receive the necessary vitamins and minerals to maintain health. In addition, large amounts of alcohol hinders or completely stops the digestion of food, since alcohol reduces the secretion of digestive enzymes of the pancreas. Alcohol also prevents the transport of nutrients in the blood. These disorders of digestion and absorption for a long period of time can lead to malnutrition.

Alcohol - is a universal poison that destroys all the systems and organs. With the growth of permanent intoxication, the person loses all sense of proportion and control of alcohol consumed. As a result of damaged central nervous system that leads to psychosis and neuritis.

The entire population can be divided into the following groups:

People who do not consume alcohol at all

People who use alcohol in moderation

People who abuse alcohol

In turn, the group of people who abuse alcohol, can be divided into 3 classes:

Persons who are not ill with chronic alcoholism.

Persons who develop symptoms of chronic alcoholism.

Individuals who are suffering from chronic alcoholism in the severe form.

The harm of alcoholism

The basis of any alcoholic beverage is ethyl alcohol. Ethyl alcohol itself is a highly toxic poison. Therefore, in whatever drink he may be - low-alcohol or strong, it has a detrimental effect on the internal organs of the body. Moreover, frequent alcohol addictive organism that causes disease such as alcoholism.

Alcohol ingested, it is rapidly absorbed mucous membrane of the stomach and intestine and enters the bloodstream within 5 minutes. Through the blood alcohol enters the brain and liver, where it becomes the greatest number. The cerebral cortex begins to work less organized: impaired concentration, impaired attention, thoughts are not connected. Expanding the capillaries under the skin, due in increased blood flow to the skin, which leads to the sensation of heat. But in fact, this feeling is deceptive, alcohol does not have a warming effect on the body. The impact on the center of the brain, which is responsible for the delayed release of urine by the kidneys, resulting in the fact that there is an acceleration of urine. The large amount of alcohol affects the cerebral cortex, so that disturbed coordination of movements, speech, behavior changes in the shortest period of time

In addition, the damaging effects of alcohol on the gastric mucosa, destroying it. Continuous destruction of the mucous leads to serious diseases of the stomach, such as an ulcer. The destruction of liver cells by the impact of alcohol on her lead to diseases such as cirrhosis and liver cancer. According to a survey of the organism of people suffering from alcoholism, it revealed that no body to which alcohol is not provided to its harmful effects. In addition, long reception of alcohol leads to a long hangover that lasts for several days and can lead to mental disorders, which is called "delirium tremens".

Causes of Alcoholism

One of the causes of alcoholism in unsecured people is the low standard of living. First of all, it is the heavy living conditions, poor nutrition, lack of cultural entertainment and a hopelessness. This is the reason of alcoholism. However, there is a pattern of many modern developed countries that alcoholism is growing along with the growth of economic prosperity.

Drunken alcoholism - is primarily a disease of the soul! Yearning soul - that's the beginning of drunkenness. And the longing of the soul begins with the awareness of total solitude. Sometimes it takes place unconsciously. Binge alcoholism precedes usually between neuroses, phobias affect. Man is not yet aware of the reasons for their constant concern and dissatisfaction with life everlasting. First dreams blow up his mind at night. Vivid, disturbing dreams - the first symptom of the disease of loneliness.

Man is not yet aware that he is alone everywhere - in the family, at work, in a crowded park in the crowded arena of the stadium. Timeless nostalgia starts to undermine it. Big City - this cluster alone. Metro, especially in the morning - a vivid example. Come back barefoot or wearing pajamas the night, and no one will pay attention to you. Each absorbed their own loneliness.

And as long as people will come up against a desperate loneliness in the diverse, vibrant, bustling city, it will return to its own staff, have split personalities. And in this group, where he himself and himself drinking buddy, it becomes comfortable. He is getting warmer. This team of his inner world understand it, accept it, he is not alone. You just need to drink to sincere dialogue started a few individuals within the man himself. Hangover returns it in this hearty company in an alien, hostile world of complex realities. Realities ashamed of it. The evidence to him that he nothingness. And he returns to his company. This condition is called alcoholic depression.

Signs and symptoms of alcoholism

As already stated above, almost every modern man at least occasionally, but drink alcohol. However, not all alcoholics are considered - because of occasional reception of ethanol. The main and fundamental difference between a healthy person suffering from alcoholism - a relationship first - psychological, and then - physical.

The external signs of the presence of this disease in humans include:

Stay socially nigredo (low level of social well-being due to lack of desire or ability to earn money with their work);

the drunken periods (unsystematic alcohol consumption for more than one calendar day)

increase in the threshold of rejection of alcohol, no vomiting at high doses of alcohol;

increase tolerance to ethyl alcohol;

the presence of withdrawal syndromes (in other words, a hangover);

JavaScript external pathologies characterized by the complex skin aging, an increase in small veins and bruising due to micro-breaks capillaries.

Those who are exposed to alcoholism in the most advanced stages, almost out of the intoxication, completely losing their own social values and outlook. This inveterate alcoholics become incoherent and incomprehensible due to damage nerve tissue at the cellular level and impaired motor muscles. Very often drinking causes the development of cancer of the digestive tract, liver cirrhosis or liver cancer, and cardiovascular disease (often leading to death).

There is no objective explanation of the fact why modern society is drowning in rivers of alcohol that are tightened like a whirlpool of healthy people in their arms, making them virtually disabled. After all, with relatively intact functioning of organs and systems people are not able to independently give an account of their actions, dropping out of the dense structure of society.

This is especially true with regard to female alcoholism. Why is that, in recent years, this kind of disease began its epidemic spread. This fact can not but acclaim, as it is a perfect half of mankind is a basic element of any of the cells of society around which all revolves. It is necessary to realize this and to make every effort to eliminate alcohol as the main destroyer of women's lives.

Description of the disease

Female alcoholism - a psycho-narcological disease associated with abnormal addiction to alcohol women and their systematic use, accompanied by lesions of brain tissue and internal organs. It would seem, why not? All drink alcohol and no trouble is not happening. But there are some features that are associated with the female body, and addiction to alcohol in general.

It should not be drinking alcohol periodic drinks containing alcohol in its composition. It can only be called a dangerous abuse of these substances, especially in large quantities.

Normally, the human body needs a certain amount of ethanol, which is due to the proper organization of metabolism produced daily. At the same time the female body does not hurt to 50 milliliters of alcohol equivalent to 40-50% alcohol solution that neutralizes the liver without consequences.

However, if such a model the situation in which the blood flow is systematically ethanol, even in this amount, a certain part will penetrate the blood-brain barrier is the brain. This is bound to cause irritation of the opioid receptors, which are responsible for the formation, depending on the substance. Therefore, the disease comes from far away, walking the fine line of norm and pathology.

With the development of addiction to alcohol increases the dose, regularly ingested, which has a toxic effect on the liver cells, heart, brain, kidneys, and nervous tissue. Sooner or later it will lead to irreversible structural rearrangements with the development of organ failure, which further exacerbate the toxic effects on the brain.

Features of woman alcoholism

The general laws of development of the disease in the female and male body are no different. But there are some features that made highlight female alcoholism separate disease. It is characterized by its own laws affecting development, for, consequences and treatment of problems. These include:

Relative psycho-emotional lability women. This means that their higher nervous activity arranged in the predominance not logical, and intuitive operation of the brain. In this regard, they are more emotional and more exposed to the negative effects of stress factors;

Increased sensitivity of liver tissue to the toxic effects of ethanol on the background of reducing the ability of the enzyme systems for processing and disposal. This results in a duration of action of small doses and it severely damaged liver cirrhosis transformation;

The fragile structure of nerve cells and interneuronal connections. This leads to disruption of neurotransmission at the early stages of alcoholism in women;

Slow blood flow in the depot organs. These are the liver and spleen. This is due to the relatively low metabolic activity, hypotension (low blood pressure), and a large volume of veins, which further contributes to the damage of these organs;

The weak structure of the blood-brain barrier (special membrane that limits the brain from toxic substances). As a result of this particular drink falls almost freely in unprotected neurons;

Reduced secretory function of the skin and kidneys, which slows down the excretion of metabolic products of ethanol;

Rapid absorption in the intestine;

Incompatibility between female hormones and degradation products of alcohol.

Thus, there is a situation that the woman herself is not aware of it very early starts to feel the need for alcohol. It very quickly causes a decrease in self-criticism, and any comments about this family, are denied. Even faster the damage to the brain, liver and other internal organs. Ultimately, all at lightning speed results in a severe form of alcohol dependence and the reception of multiple organ dysfunction.

Signs and symptoms of female alcoholism

It is unlikely that the woman who is drawn into a dangerous disease, will be able to identify at its signs. The main responsibility lies with her loved ones. Especially if they are the right way of life. Of course, if there are "associates" living according to the laws of alcohol dependence, to realize the disease will not be possible at all. These people are really unhappy, as they lose everything without realizing it. When thinking - it appears that time has been lost. Therefore, it is important to note female alcoholism is still in its infancy. Its symptoms include:

The increased desire for consumption of alcoholic beverages, no matter what. Sick alcoholism, begin to look for any reason and an excuse to drink;

The categorical denial of the comments in their direction about alcohol abuse;

Increasing doses of alcohol needed to achieve intoxication, was not there before;

Rejection of "biting" After the adoption of servings of beverages containing ethanol, and loss of appetite in general;

Loss of interest in the hobby and values that occurred before;

Closure of person and communication with people with alcohol dependence;

Inadequate behavior: rudeness, hysteria, obscene speech, which had not previously observed;

Reduced self-criticism and intelligence;

The irresponsible attitude to work and the use of funds for the purchase of alcoholic beverages;

Drinking alcohol alone;

Cyanosis and facial puffiness;

The increase in the size of the stomach due to the development of alcoholic cirrhosis of the liver;

Shiver (tremor) limbs.

These symptoms develop, depending on the stage of the disease gradually stratifying each other. The importance of their progression belongs to reduced excitability of the vomiting center in the brain. The heavier the stage, the more inhibited the gag reflex, which leads to the fact that female alcoholics with extensive clinical experience never feeling of nausea and vomiting.

Stages of female alcoholism

The clinical course of female alcoholism are three stages. Their designation is expedient in terms of dependence and complications, as well as remedial measures.

The first stage. In regard to the pathogenic, presented the process of the emergence of alcohol addiction. During this time there is an addictive opioid receptors to the products of a number of ethanol. This process paves the beginning of formation of persistent psychological dependence and transition process in the second stage. Clinically it is manifested unusual woman's desire to have a drink. Typically, this is motivated by poor health, problems in the family and at work. Most importantly, it occurs more frequently than previously observed, indicating that the failure of the brain to resist the pathological desire.

The second stage. It occurs when the opioid receptors cause irritation of the brain in the absence of alcohol. This suggests that women already have a mental dependence on it. Structural changes in the neurons of the brain tissue and internal organs missing. Clinical manifestations in this stage may take the form of drunken forms or continuous use. For women, a characteristic of the second form of the disease, leading to rapid fading of the female body and the transition process to the next step.

The third stage. It is characterized by irreversible structural changes in opioid receptors, the brain and other organs. This leads to permanent dependence on alcohol, the use of which is becoming a way of life of affected women. Thus, in addition to psychological dependence develop organ dysfunction.

Consequences of woman alcoholism

Given the fact that female alcoholism is characterized by fulminant, it very quickly leads to serious consequences. All they either violate the normal functioning or cause damage to internal organs incompatible with life. These include:

Toxic alcoholic encephalopathy in lesions of the brain;

Polyneuropathy in violation of the structure and functioning of peripheral nerves;

Critical reduction of intelligence and mental disabilities;

Delirium tremens (white garyachka);

Toxic hepatitis with transformation into cirrhosis and portal hypertension with the development of ascites;

Overdose and poisoning alcohol substitutes;

Renal insufficiency;

Acute and chronic pancreatitis, pancreatic necrosis (damage to the pancreas);

Position of compression syndrome that occurs when women get drunk to the point where they do not feel anything peredavlivayut segments extremities. Thus, there is poor circulation in them, resulting in gangrene with subsequent amputation.

Increased risk of heart attacks and strokes.

How to cure a female alcoholism?

How to cure a female alcoholism

In deciding whether to help women suffering from alcoholism, should be guided by the most important rule: "the rescue of drowning - the handiwork of drowning." As much as it may sound cruel, but in fact and situation. If a woman does not realize that she got off from the correct way of life, yielding to evil influence, no effect of the most expensive methods of treatment can be expected.

Therefore, such a person must be surrounded by the necessary attention. A woman should feel that she is full and someone needs it. But it is not worth much to load it with all sorts of problems, especially when the motivation for treatment. You can never put pressure on such a person. All arguments and observations need to try to cause mild. Patience - that what you need to stock up on all the loved ones. The only way to force a man to come to an understanding of the problem.

When this happens, you can not lose a single day. Women should be patient substance abuse hospital, where it will be carried out comprehensive treatment.

Specialized psychological and psychotherapeutic help.

Detoxification therapy.

Drug treatment of alcoholism itself - drugs, forming an aversion to alcohol in women (disulfiram).

Suturing of alcoholism - subcutaneous administration of drugs that block the opioid receptors in the brain (naltrexone). Depending on the dose depends on the validity of the drug.

Coding with the help of hypnosis and psychotherapy.

Correction of pathology of the internal organs.

Consistent and phased implementation of each of the treatment depends on the stage of alcoholism and is subject to strict individual selection. It is not necessary to postpone it. After all, nothing in life happens for a reason.

Teenage alcoholism - is one form of intoxication. It is characterized by addiction to alcohol. It can develop in patients of different age groups, regardless of gender and social status. This disease has the ability to cause addiction in people with no established mentality - for example, in adolescents.

On the disease indicates a reaction to the fact of refusal of alcohol. If this happens, among adolescents in a patient who developed an addiction manifest:

Irritability.

Discontent.

Viciousness

In the absence of intervention, notably the state of discomfort. On the formation of abuse said receiving frequency and decreasing the importance of reason. At the same time increases the amount received. The body of a teenager habitually drinking there is a need to adapt to the effects of alcohol.

His normal condition allows him to produce new cells. When addiction to alcohol slows this natural ability. Instead, the body has to take care of the security measures for the processing of large servings of alcohol that must be neutralized when it enters the body. The ability to cope with the load is gradually reduced, and there comes a stage of alcohol poisoning.

Alcohol is bad for any patient. Adolescents disappears ability to refrain from sexual desire. Early onset of sexual activity leads to the depletion of certain stock diagnosed overvoltage neuro-genital area. Due to the use of alcohol by teenagers awaken sexual desire, whether prosperous circumstances.

In such a side effect is a consequence - together with alcohol it causes weakening of sexual function at an early age. There are many consequences of alcoholism and adolescence, he often ends the decline of fertility.

Causes of alcoholism in teenagers

Teenage Alcoholism

Causes of alcoholism in teenagers are divided into two groups. They laid in psychology, heredity and other factors. A common reason to consider:

Trying to stick to traditions.

Meet sensations.

To overcome shyness and some complexes in communication.

Find an understanding with others.

Teenagers think that alcohol - this is an excellent means to open up, a kind of pathogen, which can not be much harm. When you first experience it appears that due to alcohol:

there is bitterness,

a burning sensation in the mouth,

heavier head, pains begin.

The most difficult time he decides not to use alcohol. But each time the discomfort seem normal to them the habit.

The complexities of the disease associated with many reasons to drink. Even patients who do not lead an active life with constant achievements, forced to celebrate:

end of school,

admission to college or university,

device part time,

Birthdays.

Produced habit. In adults, there is a sense of the everyday life of boredom and an inability to find something to do, spend energy for logical purposes. There is a place for so-called second group of motives.

Find a good beer is a lot easier than - really worthwhile book. It is not surprising to develop appropriate preferences. Sport - a good time, but it needs power, requires a very strong stimulus, a certain state of health. Moreover, at first glance it seems that alcohol is cheaper than lessons in good company. Apparently have a negative impact media, as well - the same books and movies where alcohol justify as normal in the fashion glamorous life.

Statistics alcoholism among teenagers

Statistics alcoholism among adolescents was important in the world. Based on the data obtained in the US succeeded in obtaining certain figures. Examined data reports American drug treatment. Without exception, all studies show: in different states 90-92% of children in the age group 14 - 18 years time to try alcohol. With increasing age of the test increases the number of doses. The Swiss Institute for the fight against alcoholism conducted a lot of research, touching almost all European countries. They tried to establish the reasons for which minors younger individuals there drinking. Responses showed that:

61% of all - because I like it, gives a certain pleasure;

23% - to look like other drinkers in the company;

16% - in order to relax, to muscle tension.

The first trial of alcoholic beverages accounted for 10 - 13 years. To develop the habit requires 2 years. First, the aim is to relax, have a good time, feel deceptive introduction to adulthood.

Age of alcoholism continues to get younger. While the peak of mass initiation and acquisition of habit are aged 14-15 years. These patients are accustomed to massively use drugs ..

The consequences of teenage alcoholism

The consequences associated with adolescent alcoholism that at this age the body is under development. At this age, there comes a stage of growth and development of the major organ systems and functions. The impact of alcohol on their ends with serious illnesses and incurable pathologies.

Of particular danger are the consequences for the psyche. In ordinary cases, teenager unable to return to normal. To form itself requires time that this age has not yet been formed. It occurs only in adulthood.

Most complications occur in adolescents:

mental deterioration,

various emotional disorders and volitional

reduced mental activity,

it is impossible to work normally,

constantly changing mood,

Normal sleep is broken,

spoils the character, develop the quality of the worst teen,

the immune system is exposed to negative changes,

endocrine organs and nervous system are deformed,

derange the functioning of the respiratory, digestive, urinary system,

constantly felt tired,

after a day of load power can not be restored.

At the most severe disease occurs death.

Prevention of teenage alcoholism

Prevention of teenage alcoholism is largely connected with psychology. Age comes a time when a person's personality is formed, and - his body, health, and others. This time is not desirable to use harmful substances that can lead to intoxication. Among these compositions - alcohol and alcoholic beverages.

Under the influence of alcohol the body is exposed to harmful. For prevention of this disease it is necessary to start from an early age, starting with the psychological approach. The basis for it are measures that help to form a correct picture of the danger.

It is important that a person with a properly formed mental and physical point of view. We need to find ways to take the teenager on his spare time, encouraged his passion, to develop the desire to learn and succeed as adults.

It is important to detect the disease if stepped alcoholism. Treatment should be done at the medical profession, this will help avoid a relapse and achieve the desired result.

Children's alcoholism - a complex psychological and physiological dependence, is detrimental to the health of the growing organism, and the risk of complete degradation increases markedly. Regardless of the factors such as social, in the fight against this problem is no effective means. Society's views on alcohol are largely based on the fact that its presence is unavoidable, try to see it in the pros, and this attitude to a negative phenomenon affects the child's mind and perception.

Children who consistently consume alcohol, are rapidly gaining the proper relationship. To do this, they just get drunk 3-4 times per month. Negative changes occur:

It slows the growth function.

Personality degraded.

Quickly there is a dependence on alcohol.

In the psyche of violations occur.

Destroys the internal organs.

Sexual development goes wrong or slows down.

In children, these processes occur much more quickly than adults or adolescents. Children of alcoholics are transformed into very quickly. This bad habit as alcoholism, is a kind of substance abuse.

Children's alcoholism

Statistics shows that the process of alcohol abuse in 75% of cases develop up to 20 years. 46% of the cases include adolescence. Growth of the disease in Russia particularly covers adolescence. The results of the statistics and surveys have shown that 56% of those studying in classes 8-10, drinks tasted bad, and the majority of students 12-13 years old already have experience using and even - the purchase of this product.

Only 6% of the total number of high school students have resisted the temptation, the rest are drinking harmful drink with the regularity of a different sort. About 30% of young people do it every week. It is - quite dismal performance, they say that the risk of developing dependence increases all the time.

Diagnosis is made to set several parameters. Among them:

Upon receipt of alcohol disappears emetic response.

Lack of control over the volume of alcohol consumed.

Retrograde amnesia in partial form.

The development of withdrawal symptoms.

Binge drinking binge type.

At the same time dramatically lowers the level of the average age of minors who abuse alcohol. Now he has reached 14 - 11 years. They are dominated by beer drinkers.

Causes of child alcoholism

Causes of child alcoholism is largely based on psychology. Children's kind of them include the following:

lack of attention on the part of adults and parents;

undue pressure from the parents;

thus attempt to move away from problems;

the proximity of the corresponding example, such as drinking parents;

attempt to assert itself, is a misconception that it makes the child an adult;

bad influence of the company;

the excess of free time.

The problems mentioned above relate to children and adolescent alcoholism. The majority of this category habit habits appear literally in the womb, if a woman dares to alcohol. Alcohol has the ability to be provided in fetal blood, penetrating to the placenta. Develops risk of fatal alcohol syndrome. Appear related symptoms, among them - the anomalies of the maxillofacial region:

the elongated shape of the face,

zygomatic arch with hypoplasia,

low forehead,

hypoplasia of the bone of the chin,

wrong mandible

deformed thorax, insufficient length of the feet, weak extension of the elbow joints, abnormal location of the fingers, hips underdeveloped,

strabismus, narrow eye slits form, the upper eyelid is omitted,

often sealed neck, the head grows a little,

too small nose, with a saddle type, with a short nasal bridge,

shortened upper lip, "harelip" pathological structure of the sky - the so-called "Palate"

low birth weight,

physical development goes wrong,

delayed growth, or, on the contrary, is excessively high,

nervous system develops properly diagnosed microcephaly (underdevelopment of the brain)

heart defects, disorders genital-anal value, genitals and joints.

In the habit of visiting many causes and risk factors. It is believed that social status has little effect on the values of the harmful addiction. But in poor families, in a lower standard of living, such habits appear spontaneously appear one of the signs belonging to the most poor strata of society. At high risk of prosperity no less great. Slightly better things with good genetics, but in this case there is a danger. It is advisable to show the life of a child with a good hand, avoiding the bad companies, feasts in the family circle, notations. Also, it makes no sense to read the rules of the child that adults do not observe - in this case, will not help any arguments.

Heredity - quite a complex science. Genetics operates with a fact: the genes determining susceptibility to irrevocably drunkenness does not exist. It is responsible for this large group of factors. It is always possible to inculcate a child the habit all have an opinion, to judge the situation adequately.

Consequences of child alcoholism

Consequences of child alcoholism irrevocably different, because health will never become standard. Among the dangerous prospects:

gastrointestinal disorders - their appearance causes the inability of children to have a snack. They usually drink in secret, eating at one time a very big portions. This carries the risk of gastritis, an inflammation of the esophagus. Very developing liver disease, pancreas;

manifest disease of the cardiovascular system, diagnosed tachycardia, varicose veins, and blood pressure rises, there is an arrhythmia, myocardial etc .;

immunity significantly reduced;

constant state of vitamin deficiency;

It can be said about the dangerous and irreversible consequences of child alcoholism - violation of brain functions, as well as in the central nervous system to lockup common development, levels of intelligence, memory, logic, and the decline of abstract forms of thinking. Personality irreversibly degraded develop incurable mental disorders.

Prevention of child alcoholism

Prevention of child alcoholism required in full. Alcoholism is a very dangerous kind of addiction. It includes a set of bad habits, the base of which - the alcohol. As a result of significantly deteriorating health, way of life is reduced. It destroys the functioning of the body. Pathogenic effects very much.

It is necessary to prevent the disease, beginning with prevention. Prevention of child alcoholism and includes factors such protection:

happy family;

material prosperity;

Training adoption of social norms;

regular medical examinations;

dwelling in the safe area;

a sufficient level of self-esteem;

production should have a positive character traits.

Prevention of child alcoholism is to eliminate risk factors and strengthening protective factors.

Early diagnosis of alcoholism in a child can quickly recover, with appropriate measures. It is important to take care of a competent prevention, to provide children with an opportunity to find a good hobby - hiking in the section, study and others. From the need to achieve the elimination of alcohol from the market, to make it clear that one can live without this product. When conscientious objection adult alcohol alcoholism children will decline and will cease to provide a risk.

Beer alcoholism - a term that refers to the painful craving for beer. This concept is not an official diagnosis, but the severity of the problem is not removed. Abuse of a beer is not regarded as a separate species of alcoholism, but is perceived as a quick way to alcohol dependence. Feature beer alcoholism is that it is evolving rapidly, and gradually, as the beer is considered to be harmless, and many low-alcohol drinks are not considered seriously. Such an attitude towards this drink for the following reasons:

Advertisement forms the idea of beer as a companion easy, successful life, indispensable attribute of intimate gatherings and feasts;

Society sees a man with a bottle of beer quietly drinking it is not aware of the dangers in full;

The drink has some really relaxing effect and quite pleasant taste.

Beer alcoholism many consider less harmful to health than others of his species. Meanwhile, it spreads rapidly, the number of sufferers from this disease is huge, and they do not believe that they need treatment.

To determine the presence of such a diagnosis in the early stages is very difficult to later appear more clearly indicators painful craving for beer.

Signs and symptoms of the beer alcoholism

Beer alcoholism

Signs of alcohol dependence beer are similar to "vodka" alcoholism because it's not the drink, and alcohol, which it contains. But patients with this diagnosis at the time of referral to a specialist are usually heavier and running the form, which is characterized by the following features:

loose body;

overweight;

noisy, heavy breathing;

eye bags;

cyanotic complexion;

unrecoverable peculiar smell soaked apples or acetone, which constitutes a violation of the functions of the pancreas, as well as an increased level of sugar.

Moreover, such patients complain JavaScript weakness, shortness of breath, pain in the lumbar region and the right hypochondrium. There has been a sharp decrease in potency, or lack thereof, there are problems with fertilization.

Under the influence of beer male hormone - testosterone - is no longer produced, and it is replaced by a female, which leads to an increase in male breast, pelvis and expansion of excess adiposity.

Symptoms of psychological dependence are:

need to increase the dose of beer to get the initial effect of its impact;

frequent use of the drink in large quantities;

the lack of beer causes irritation, aggressiveness;

intoxication is accompanied by loss of memory;

lost control of the situation, the person starts to drink beer, regardless of location, time, and the company;

Night insomnia is replaced by daytime sleepiness;

there is a desire in the morning hangover;

I can not relax, lift your mood without beer;

it is impossible to reduce the volume of drink and it exceeds a liter per day.

Match more than two points is a signal to the possible presence of disease.

Hangover from drinking beer similar to the ordinary, but to get rid of its manifestations is much more difficult. Here are some of them:

persistent diarrhea;

low levels of well-being;

severe headaches.

For beer alcoholism is not characterized by periods of binge, but the patient is applied to the bottle several times a day, so the state does not manage to come sober, therefore, weeks, months, and sometimes years, these people are intoxicated.

The consequences of beer alcoholism

Beer has on the terrible devastating effect. According to hazard it can be compared only to that of moonshine, as soon as they are during alcoholic fermentation is stored in full with alcohol related toxic compounds: fusel oils, aldehydes, methanol, ether. It's worth noting that beer can contain up to 14% alcohol, so it is not always wise to consider low-alcohol drinks. Habituation is developing three times faster than when using other alcohol, and psychological man did not feel the danger, and not struggling with addiction.

The effects of systematic drinking beer affects all areas of the body:

Heart - this body is greatly increased in size at the beer alcoholism, there is even a special term: "Bavarian heart," he means that the heart cavity wall and widened thicker steel, developed in cardiac muscle necrosis, mitochondria decreased. This effect is due to the high concentration of cobalt exceeds the norm by 10 times. Negative impact on the work of the heart received a large amount of alcohol and carbonation. Once in the body, beer literally overwhelms the bloodstream, causing varicose veins and heart borders. Appears syndrome "nylon stocking" in which the heart muscle is greatly increased in size, it becomes flabby, sagging worse pumps blood.

The brain - the brain cells from dying because of alcohol, into the blood, and then the kidneys and excreted in the urine. When the beer alcoholism devastating effect, even more than when exposed to vodka because beer, among other harmful substances, there is similarity ptomaine - cadaverine. The systematic use of beer reduces the learning person IQs fall. Without proper treatment of beer drinking is fraught with decline in personal assessment and dementia.

Nervous system - the beer is different in that it contains some psychoactive substances capable of creating lightweight mind-numbing effect. Consequently, a person is exposed not only to the effects of alcohol, but also sedatives. Over time, it is impossible without the beer to relax and calm down. Doses of consumption are growing, there are alcoholic excesses, deteriorating memory. Narcologists equate beer to drugs and noted his aggressiveness, which explains the numerous examples of complete beer gatherings killing, fighting, looting and rape.

Hormones - toxic substances and heavy metals contained in beer, change the endocrine system. Suppresses the production of testosterone in men, it leads to the feminization of the male population. Fat accumulates on the thighs, hips, breast cancer grow, expanding hips. Women often drink beer, are at risk of infertility or cancer. They coarsens his voice and appear "beer mustache." If the beer is to drink breast-feeding her child can begin epileptic seizures.

Reproductive function - beer alcoholism provokes changes in the testes and ovaries. Regenerate seminiferous tubules and connective tissues grow testicular parenchyma. Toxic effects on the adrenal glands inhibits the production of androgens, which are responsible for sexual desire, it comes as a result of the reduction or complete absence.

Gastrointestinal apparatus - its components are in constant tension, especially in the liver. Regular beer consumption leads to weakening of the barrier infection, the emergence of foci of inflammation and cirrhosis. "Palpable liver" - one of the most frequent diagnoses associated beer alcoholism. Ethyl alcohol is irritating to mucous membranes, provokes inflammation and gastritis. Gastric mechanisms of self-defense are trying to cope with the situation and produce more mucus until until atrophy. As a result of impaired digestion, food stagnates or is not ready in the intestines, causing severe pain. It is proved that beer consumption promotes the development of colon cancer.

Kidneys - the beer has a pronounced diuretic effect and contributes to leaching from the body of nutrients: protein, minerals (magnesium, potassium, vitamin C) and fat, carbohydrates. This leads to numerous health problems. Disturbed under the influence of beer and acid-base balance, which causes the kidneys to work in emergency mode. This situation leads to the fact that renal vessels become thinner and there is a risk of hemorrhage in the kidney.

How to get rid of the beer alcoholism?

Getting rid of the hard drive to the beer. This is due to the fact that beer drinking can be considered "polunarkomaniey" because of the content in the drink drugs. Therefore, the amount of necessary aid to the patient increases, required course treatment.

Beer alcoholism is usually formed at a young age, when the mechanisms of co-dependence is very strong, requiring the intervention of a specialist to correct them.

Treatment of beer depending aims to eliminate the main symptoms, namely:

excretion of excess fluid;

stimulation of damaged organs;

introduction of detoxification solutions.

Get rid completely of beer alcoholism can only with the support of the patient and the therapist psychiatrist.

Medicines that would treat alcoholism, but there are drugs used to combat addiction. They are divided into those that cause alcohol intolerance, reduce the drive or facilitate the hangover.

The main stage on the road to recovery - the awareness of having problems of dependence. Then the person should look for a way to stop drinking beer.

Sometimes it is a willful decision, backed by understanding the magnitude of threat. If this method did not prove, you can try to reduce the dose. Only need to do it consistently and rigorously.

Drink beer is often associated with a certain ritual, habit, way of life, so we need to change it. For example, those who are used to spend evenings at home in front of the TV with a beer drink, it is worth trying to take the evening with something else, such as walking around the city, sauna, or classes at the fitness club. The change of surroundings will help to distract from the need to take alcohol

An additional motivation can become a cash consideration when a person throws each day in the treasury the amount that is usually spent on beer. And six months later It can be purchased for these funds some useful and coveted thing, or go on vacation.

Along with these methods is to seek professional help, it can help solve the problem in the complex and in a shorter time.

Beer alcoholism - a dangerous disease that is a long time to diagnose and is not recognized by the patient, it causes serious disturbances in the body, and then it is difficult to be treated and is fraught with serious complications.

Prevention of Alcoholism

Under the prevention of alcoholism understand such methods, which are aimed at the formation of a negative attitude towards alcohol. The main objective is to create a way of life in man, which he will not have the craving for alcohol. There are three stages of prevention of alcoholism.

Traditional medicine can cure many diseases, which are not always good at modern medicine. For example, treatment of epilepsy, the treatment of myocardial infarction folk remedies are not seldom give greater effect but we'll talk about the book See the following. Traditional medicine includes treatments for their systematic and long-term effects on the body composition, which are beneficial for the body components. Their impact is not limited to a certain organ. There is an impact on the whole body. This is the best healing, so one does not have separate bodies of non-interacting with each other.

Primary prevention of alcoholism

Primary prevention is aimed at preventing the occurrence of alcoholism. Such actions are usually directed to the story, about the harmful effects of alcohol. That as a result a person has formed an alternative life in which alcohol will not play any role. It is proved that the best method of prevention of alcoholism, is the formation of the consciousness of human personality so that alcohol is no longer a value in life.

The consequences of alcohol abuse are devastating: broken families, mangled fate, children with disabilities, increased criminal activity in the soil and drinking more. Diseases that brings with it the inability to cope with alcohol craving - rectal cancer, nervous disorders, gastrointestinal problems, alcoholic hepatitis and pancreatitis, cirrhosis, genetic diseases and mental ... Russian official statistics, only losing a year to 600 thousand people due to alcohol deaths but the real figure is very likely much more.

In addition we must remember that "a little bit" - is not considered. Usually beer craving for alcohol is not limited to: cocktails, wine, fortified wine, liqueurs, vodka, brandy - the "noble" long drinks waiting for their turn. "Americanization" way of life imposed on them Russians, some unusual alcoholic habits. For example, a glass of wine for breakfast, lunch and dinner; business lunches with libations; corporate events; brasseries without appetizers; restaurant alcohol "etiquette." Not surprisingly, among the recognized medicine alcoholics turned out famous faces of culture, art, politics, show business and the business world. Not so long ago, even the first President of Russia has been linked with numerous scandals alcohol - not to mention the less significant figures?

Secondary prevention of alcoholism

Secondary prevention is aimed at the treatment of patients already alcoholism. This program includes work with the family of the patient, his meeting with former alcoholics, interview and broad social and psychological assistance.

Alcoholism is insidious in that its effect on humans strictly individually: the habit of ethyl alcohol formed under the influence of a combination of factors. This genetic predisposition, and the impact of their own social group with his opinions and traditions, and mental instability, etc. It is noted that female alcoholism is less common men, but the disease is more negative consequences. And, importantly, the later stages of alcoholism virtually untreatable - akin to substance abuse. Yes, and how many want him to be treated? Especially because the law requires the voluntary consent of the patient to treatment. Meanwhile, the transition from one stage to the next identified a complex way, and the patient, considering that always stay, often misses the "point of return."

Tertiary prevention of alcoholism

Tertiary prevention aims to help people recovering from alcoholism. This program includes psychological counseling and attending Alcoholics Anonymous.

Closing

As with any other disease, it is necessary to carry out prevention of alcoholism. Alcoholism is better to prevent than to face them as a result of crises in life.

Well, dear druzbya now I'll tell you a few secrets how to save people from addiction.

Treatment of alcoholism without the knowledge of the patient.

The method is quite specific, but it is very effective and is targeted only for the treatment of alcoholism without the knowledge of the patient. Aversion to alcohol will last from several weeks to several months. For this catch 15-30 green bugs. They can be found on raspberry bushes. And immediately put them in vodka volume of 0.5 liters.

After 2-3 days vodka infusions, and you can give it to the patient to drink. Suffice it to '50 only to the patient does not have to say anything about it.

Unctuously salt from alcoholism

Elaine G - the so-called living stone. This is - a unique product, it is permitted to give the drinker when he does not know. This natural product was known in Russia in the era of Ivan the Terrible. Unusual ingredients found in the VII century, along with the mines of the Volga region. It is believed that a substance known today gave his father Nestor serving rector of Old Believers in Sukhodolskiy monastery of the Holy Trinity. Unctuous Salt, father Nestor transmitted to people who successfully struggles with alcohol dependence, and its use is very simple.

"Unctuous salt" is a component in the creation of church incense and substance - olive oil, which includes incense. It is a dry extract of herbs "Perun semitsvet" family of thyme.

Hangover can be removed if it is correct to treat the formation of anti-alcoholic reflex. Alcohol should become a contradiction that is best achieved without the knowledge of the patient.

Recipe: In the fight against drunkenness use the following recipe. A portion of the salt (30g - 1 tablespoon uppers) are dissolved in 100 g. pharmacy alcohol, the mixture is then necessary to insist 3 days, choosing to place a dark place. The patient should drink 7 drops of the day when they are dissolved in a drink or food. Time of day usage - does not matter.

Treatment of alcoholism dung fungus

The fungus beetle

It is common fungi that eat each. Mushroom caps - 3-7 cm in diameter, at first ovate, gray-brown, darker in the center, with small brown scales. The recipe is intended for the treatment of alcoholism without the knowledge of the patient. You can cook the mushrooms and fry as you please, but do not eat them together with alcohol. When used dung mushrooms together with alcohol poisoning of the body takes place. And the mushrooms and the procedure is absolutely safe for human drinking.

Another advantage is that the fungus remains in effect for a few days. Therefore, if the next day the man again drink a glass or two, the symptoms will return with the same force.

Treatment of alcoholism infusion of thyme

The herb thyme

When used infusion of herbs thyme together with alcohol, a strong nausea and vomiting. And it can be added directly into the bottle to the patient himself did not know. To prepare this infusion, pour 3 tablespoons of thyme in a glass. Pour the boiling water and cover. A few hours later the grass is ready. Take one tablespoon 2 times a day. After drinking some vodka, will be sufficient to 15-20 ml. Emetic response and slack stomach pain manifested in half an hour. Treatment is carried out daily during the week. But without the combination with alcohol treatment lasts a month.

Treatment of infusion of red pepper

Tested national treatment of alcoholism without the knowledge of a tincture of red peppers. For its preparation take half a liter of 60% alcohol, and to sprinkle one tablespoon of red pepper powder. After 2 weeks, the medication is ready. Add 2-3 drops of the tincture per liter of alcohol.

List of herbs that help to recover from alcoholism.

Ivan tea (tea Koporye) alcoholism

Many people know that such Indian tea, Chinese tea, but few know that there is also a Russian tea or Koporye tea, also known as Ivan the tea. This traditional drink has a very long history that dates back to the 12th century and was once known worldwide.

Hard to believe, but the Russian Koporye tea or tea is made in very large quantities and was very common to all the world, especially in England. The mention of the Russian tea is found in the English encyclopedia, records dated to the 18th century. It was exported to many countries, and by sales ahead of hemp, gold and fur. After the First World War trade in tea it was stopped, and after the revolution production was stopped altogether.

The popularity of tea causes its composition. Ivan tea - herb, has long been known for its beneficial properties. Ivan tea is included in the leaders on the content of vitamin C and vitamin P, boosts immunity, strengthens blood vessels, removes toxins and heavy metals. Another useful feature of Ivan-tea is its ability to help in various intoxications and poisonings, with radiation damage. It perfectly cleanses the body, including for alcohol poisoning. Koporye tea increases efficiency.

Ivan tea or tea Koporye useful in endocrine disorders, and inflammatory processes in the body. Another special feature of Russian tea is the ability to increase potency, to help in the treatment of BPH and prostatitis.

Ivan tea against alcohol, prescription. To reduce the craving for alcohol and to remove hangover willow-herb should be mixed with thyme in a ratio of 5: 1 and brew. Drink with honey when a craving for alcohol. Throughout the day to drink 5-7 cups of tea.

Hellebore water (puppeteer grass) from alcoholism

Hellebore Lobel know under the name of the puppeteer (grass). In nature, a perennial herb can reach over a meter in height. He laid a lot of useful features, including quite significant:

analgesic,

antiparasitic,

antimycotic.

This is a very poisonous plant! The largest number of the poison - at its root, as well as the rootstock, so do not try to prepare it yourself!

Hellebore water - known medical cure. His purchase without providing recipes in almost any drugstore. 100 ml of this water contained 50 ml. tinctures, created on the roots and rhizomes of hellebore, plus 50 ml of purified water. This tool is now used in folk medicine and its main direction - the fight against parasites in the human body.

Due to its composition, this water worsens the state of drunk. On the one hand, begins the conclusion of toxins and poisons. On the other - a feeling not want to experience once again. Thus, alcoholics created a negative attitude towards alcohol. It is no more give satisfaction as before, and the alcoholic begins to feel bad feeling after drinking only vodka, without the addition of the drug. All the same painful symptoms appear, such as:

severe nausea,

vomiting,

loose stools,

heart failure in the acute form,

severe cramping,

increased muscle tone,

sneezing,

weakness with trembling.

Kpyten European alcoholism

Kopytnik Europe has many advantages. This is an unusual plant with a green leaves with a smooth shiny surface. The medicinal properties of the rhizome is used, and - the very roots. To treat alcoholism, they are collected when it is the second half of the summer, or - in the autumn. It is advisable to use fresh components. Dry fragments can be in a room that is well ventilated.

Always worth to consult a doctor!

Recipe 1: a teaspoon of root, finely chopped, pour a glass of boiling water. It must insist in a pot with a tight lid. After 3-4 hours, you can use the liquid. The pre-filter it. Then the patient must drink it with vodka. In the glass it is necessary to pour 1 tablespoon possible - two tablespoons of the whole bottle, mix directly into it. Because infusion induce vomiting. There are side effects - similar to those that cause the common emetics.

2. Famous Recipe recipe when plant roots are mixed with 2 teaspoons of the pericarp and the famous walnut. This mixture is used in an amount of

1 teaspoon and pour 4 liters of wine. Cooking time - 2 weeks. A serving is 1 cup, 1-2 times a day before meals. Much worse condition, the patient is forced to give up alcohol.

Side effects. Contraindicated for use without the knowledge of the exact formulation and supervision of a physician. In case of overdose noticeable irregularities in the kidney, gall bladder, liver and stomach.

Lovage root of alcoholism

Lovage root is used since ancient times. This is a known agent in herbal medicine and traditional medicine. Doctors know him as a good remedy for obesity, heart problems. In folk medicine also know that to achieve the effect it must be combined with the bay leaf. The result is called stable emetic reaction to any alcohol-based products and tools.

Tincture lovage. To prepare the desired drink - you need to take 100 grams of the roots of the plants in fresh form, as well as 10 g bay leaf, finely chop, pour a liter of vodka. For tinctures requires 3 days. The resulting drink give the patient. There is a strong emetic response within an hour.

Often enough to just smell the alcohol. The result is called aversion to any product with an appropriate composition.

Lovage enhances intestinal peristalsis. It is well suited as a nutritious food - especially for people suffering from constipation atonic. Through the course of treatment:

It stabilizes the central nervous system,

It is possible to stop a migraine,

eliminates swelling,

It acts as an anti-inflammatory.

St. John's wort for alcoholism

St. John's Wort is considered well-known folk remedy. This plant - a lot of other names:

St. John's wort,

pierced,

Punctured,

St. John's wort ordinary

It is well known for its bright yellow flowers.

A decoction of St. John's wort: 4 tablespoons herb plants in a powdered form is poured 0.5 liters of boiling water, stand with the help of a boiling water bath for 20-30 minutes, cool, strain. Reception - 2 tablespoons, twice a day, before lunch and dinner. Duration of treatment - 2 weeks. Through regular use of broth within the specified standards produced an aversion to alcohol.

A decoction of this herb is very popular. This is - a simple tool for the preparation of which need a minimum of ingredients. All are natural and safe, they do not contain alcohols and chemicals. For 2-3 weeks you can get rid of alcohol addiction.

The herb hellebore alcoholism

This herb is used in folk medicine in the fight against alcoholism. But we do not recommend it!

Dosage. The plant is by nature endowed with toxic properties. Manifestations and clinical picture in this case are similar to poisoning. When a large dose - effect dosage is too active. It is believed that this is - the reason why the hellebore does not apply traditional medicine.

There are analog, which is used externally, because a lot of hellebore medicinal properties. To get the result just two drops. They are added by pipetting, mixing with the drink, and - with food. It - instruction for a tool such as hellebore water. This is enough to irritation of the mucous airways, causing the expected reaction begins.

Overdose: Do not forget about the toxic properties of plants. Thus, in case of an overdose in the treatment of hellebore, the most innocuous symptoms of poisoning are diarrhea and vomiting. If too large a dose of hellebore drunk drugs can be fatal.

Why traditional medicine against the use of hellebore? The answer is obvious: this drug provides only topical application, but not orally (inside). Scientific studies have shown that the use of this herb man inside may lead to severe poisoning.

Thyme for alcoholism

Chabrets- one of the most popular means. It is also known as thyme.

A decoction of thyme. 15 grams of thyme brewed by the boiled water (0.5 L) was placed in a water bath for 10-15 minutes. Then the workpiece is drained, the infusion is diluted again until you reach the volume of 0.5 liters. serving 50-70 ml infusion with a little vodka (half-glasses), taken several times a day.

Quickly manifest the expected symptoms - such as nausea. The course - 1-2 weeks, many drank achieve the effect after only a few sessions. Treatment of the grass-is possible if there is the following diseases:

stomach ulcer,

thyroid disorders,

hypertonic disease,

diabetes,

bronchial asthma,

pulmonary tuberculosis.

In case of overdose experience side effects such as vomiting, which is the effect of the drug.

Tincture of thyme. For its preparation you need 3 tablespoons of raw sugar and water that is just beginning to boil. Its volume should be 200-250 ml. Time of infusion - less than an hour. The blank is necessary to drain. The daily ration is 4 tablespoons. Duration of the course - 10-14 days, then make a break for 5-7 days, and the course is repeated again.

Gathering grass exercise during flowering, waiting produced a maximum of these substances. Due to the active healing properties are produced. In this plant are particularly useful collection of leaves, flowers and shoots.

So I recommend to drink kvass (a Russian drink made of bread)

The recipe is very simple: in the three-liter capacity need 5g trembling, two loaves of bread to dry and finely chop. After cooking crumbs of black bread to pour them into the container to fill with warm water (30 degrees) to put two - three tablespoons of sugar and fill quiver. Cover with a tight lid and do not leave in a warm place for two days. After pour kvass into bottles and put on a night in the fridge. Kvass is ready can be used both during the day and at bedtime.

Warns in kvass will be about 0.1 percent alcohol so if you need to drive go first test alkotestere.

You can also order a starter for kvass from our partners write to us by e-mail. dlavrov@point-lab.ru

The cost of delivery specify in their region.

Cost for kvass leaven $ 10. - 20 liters of kvass.